Mediterran
2 Cookbooks in 1

Meditteranean Diet Vegetable Dishes + Mediterranean Salad Recipes

Table of Contents

Chapter 1.   Vegetable Dishes 3

Chapter 2.   Salad 55

Chapter 1.   Vegetable Dishes

Black Bean Stuffed Sweet Potatoes

Preparation Time: 10 minutes
Cooking Time: 40 minutes
Servings: 4
Ingredients:

- 4 sweet potatoes
- 15 ounces cooked black beans
- 1/2 teaspoon ground black pepper
- 1/2 red onion, peeled, diced
- 1/2 teaspoon sea salt
- 1/4 teaspoon onion powder
- 1/4 teaspoon garlic powder
- 1/4 teaspoon red chili powder
- 1/4 teaspoon cumin
- 1 teaspoon lime juice
- 1 1/2 tablespoons Olive oil
- 1/2 cups cashew cream sauce

Directions:

1. Spread sweet potatoes on a baking tray greased with foil and bake for 65 minutes at 350 degrees f until tender.
2. Meanwhile, prepare the sauce, and for this, whisk together the cream sauce, black pepper, and lime juice until combined, set aside until required.
3. When 10 minutes of the baking time of potatoes are left, heat a skillet pan with oil. Add in the onion to cook until golden for 5 minutes.

4. Then stir in spice, cook for another 3 minutes, stir in bean until combined, and cook for 5 minutes until hot.
5. Let roasted sweet potatoes cool for 10 minutes, then cut them open, mash the flesh, and top with bean mixture, cilantro, and avocado, and then drizzle with cream sauce.
6. Serve straight away.

Nutrition:
- Calories: 387
- Fat: 16.1 g
- Carbs: 53 g
- Protein: 10.4 g

Vegetarian Ratatouille

Preparation Time: 10 minutes

Cooking Time: 40 minutes

Servings: 4

Ingredients:

- 2 sliced red onions
- 1 sliced eggplant
- 2 sliced curettes
- 1 sliced red bell pepper
- 2 sliced squashes
- 2 cups tomato sauce
- 1/4 cups parmesan cheese
- A handful of oregano and thyme

Directions:

1. Set your oven to 375 F.
2. Stir the tomato sauce into a ceramic baking dish. Sprinkle the half of parmesan cheese over the sauce.
3. Pick one slice of each vegetable and line them up nicely. Arrange slices in a baking dish and repeat the same order. Finish with a sprinkle of remaining parmesan cheese, and herbs.
4. Cook for 35-40 minutes until the vegetables are cooked through and a little crisp.

Nutrition:

- Calories: 120
- Fats 3.5 g
- Carbs: 20 g
- Protein: 2 g

Black Bean and Quinoa Salad

Preparation Time: 10 minutes

Cooking Time: 5 minutes

Servings: 10

Ingredients:

- 15 ounces cooked black beans
- 1 chopped red bell pepper,
- 1 cup quinoa, cooked
- 1 cored green bell pepper,
- 1/2 cups vegan feta cheese

Directions:

1. In a bowl, set in all ingredients, except for cheese, and stir until incorporated. cored
2. Top the salad with cheese and serve straight away. chopped crumbled

Nutrition:

- Calories: 64
- Fat: 1 g
- Carbs: 8 g
- Protein: 3 g

Balsamic-Glazed Roasted Cauliflower

Preparation Time: 10 minutes

Cooking Time: 45 minutes

Servings: 10

Ingredients:
- 1 head cauliflower
- 1/2 pounds green beans, trimmed
- 1 peeled red onion, wedged
- 2 cups cherry tomatoes
- 1/2 teaspoon salt
- 1/4 cups brown sugar
- 3 tablespoons olive oil
- 1 cup balsamic vinegar
- 2 tablespoons chopped parsley

Directions:
1. Place cauliflower florets in a baking dish, add tomatoes, green beans, and onion wedges around it, season with salt, and drizzle with oil.
2. Pour vinegar in a saucepan, stir in sugar, bring the mixture to a boil, and simmer for 15 minutes until it is reduced by half.
3. Brush the sauce generously over cauliflower florets and then roast for 1 hour at 400°F until cooked, brushing sauce frequently. Garnish.
4. When done, garnish vegetables with parsley and then serve.

Nutrition:
- Calories: 86
- Fat: 5.7 g
- Carbs: 7.7 g
- Protein: 3.1 g

Garlicky Kale and Pea Sauté

Preparation Time: 10 minutes

Cooking Time: 8 minutes

Servings: 2

Ingredients:

- 2 sliced garlic cloves
- 1 chopped hot red chili
- 2 tablespoons olive oil
- 2 bunches chopped kale
- 1 pound frozen peas

Directions:

1. In a saucepot, mix the ingredients except for. Cook until the kale becomes tender for about 6 minutes.
2. Add peas and cook for 2 more minutes.

Nutrition:

- Calories: 85
- Fats 3 g
- Net Carbs: 11 g
- Protein: 5 g

Sun-Dried Tomato Pesto Pasta

Preparation Time: 5 minutes
Cooking Time: 11 minutes
Servings: 5
Ingredients:
- 1 cup fresh basil leaves
- 6 ounces sun-dried tomatoes
- 1 tablespoon lemon juice
- 1/2 teaspoon salt
- 1/4 cups olive oil
- 1/4 cups almonds
- 3 minced garlic cloves
- 1/2 teaspoon chopped red pepper
- 8 ounces pasta

Directions:
1. Cook the pasta according to the given ingredients instructions. For making it, toast the almonds over medium flame in a small skillet for around 4 minutes.
2. In a blender, put sun-dried tomatoes, basil, garlic, lemon juice, salt, red pepper flakes, and toasted almonds and blend it. While blending, add olive oil and blend it until it converts in the form of pesto.
3. Now coat the pasta with the pesto and serve it.

Nutrition:
- Calories: 256
- Fat: 13.7 g
- Carbs: 28.1 g
- Protein: 6.7 g

Cream Carrot Soup

Preparation Time: 5 minutes

Cooking Time: 24 minutes

Servings: 4

Ingredients:

- 1/4 teaspoon black pepper
- 1 tablespoon cilantro, chopped
- 1 onion
- 1 teaspoon turmeric powder
- 5 cups vegetable broth
- 1 pound carrots, peeled and chopped
- 2 tablespoons olive oil
- 4 celery stalks, chopped

Directions:

1. Heat up a pot with the oil over medium heat; add the onion, stir, and sauté for 2 minutes.
2. Add the carrots and the other ingredients. Bring to a simmer and cook over medium heat for 20 minutes.
3. Blend the soup using an immersion blender, ladle into bowls, and serve.

Nutrition:

- Calories: 221
- Fat: 9.6 g
- Carbs: 16 g
- Protein: 4.8 g

Lemon Arugula Salad

Preparation Time: 5 minutes
Cooking Time: 12 minutes
Servings: 5
Ingredients:

- 1 lemon
- 1/2 teaspoon sugar
- 1/2 teaspoon coarsely ground black
- 5 ounces arugula
- Pinch of pepper.
- 2 tablespoons extra virgin olive oil
- 2 ounces shaved Parmesan cheese

Directions:

1. With a paring knife, cut the top and bottom off the lemon. Cut the peel and pith away from lemon; then, into a small bowl, cut segments from between membranes. Cut each segment in half. Squeeze 1 tablespoon juice from the pulp. Sprinkle sugar over the lemon segments; let it stand for at least 10 minutes.
2. In a large bowl, mix arugula with oil, lemon segments, juice, and 1/4 teaspoon of salt.
3. Gently fold in Parmesan.
4. To serve, shave additional Parmesan on top if desired.
5. Serve immediately.

Nutrition:

- Calories: 164.3
- Fats: 15.6 g
- Net Carbs: 5.7 g
- Protein: 3.5 g

Spice-Roasted Carrots

Preparation Time: 5 minutes

Cooking Time: 45 minutes

Servings: 5

Ingredients:
- 8 large carrots
- 3 tablespoons olive oil
- 1 tablespoon red wine vinegar
- 2 tablespoons packed fresh oregano leaves
- 1 teaspoon smoked paprika
- 1/2 teaspoon ground nutmeg
- 1 tablespoon vegan butter
- Salt and pepper
- 1/3 cups salted pistachios, roasted

Directions:
1. Set your oven to 450°F.
2. Mix oregano, oil, nutmeg, paprika, carrots, salt, and pepper in a roasting pan.
3. Roast the mixture for about an hour or until the carrots become tender.
4. Transfer to a plate.
5. Top with vinegar, butter, and top with pistachios before serving.

Nutrition:
- Calories: 120
- Fats: 3.5 g
- Net Carbs: 20 g
- Protein: 2 g

Beans Salad

Preparation Time: 5 minutes
Cooking Time: 3 minutes
Servings: 16
Ingredients:
- 15 ounces green beans
- 1 pound garbanzo beans
- 15 ounces dark red kidney beans
- 1 onion
- 1/2 tablespoon white sugar
- 10 tablespoons white vinegar
- 5 tablespoons vegetable oil
- 1/2 teaspoon salt
- 1/2 teaspoon black pepper
- 1/2 teaspoon celery seed

Directions:
1. Mix all ingredients and refrigerate the salad for at least 12 hours

Nutrition:
- Calories: 126
- Fat: 8.6 g
- Carbs: 6.9 g
- Protein: 6.9 g

Grilled Zucchini with Tomato Salsa

Preparation Time: 5 minutes

Cooking Time: 10 minutes

Servings: 4

Ingredients:

- 4 zucchinis, sliced
- 1 tablespoon olive oil
- Salt and pepper
- 1 cup tomatoes, chopped
- 1 tablespoon mint, chopped
- 1 teaspoon red wine vinegar

Directions:

1. Preheat your grill.
2. Coat the zucchini with oil and season with salt and pepper.
3. Grill for 4 minutes per side.
4. Mix the remaining ingredients in a bowl.
5. Top the grilled zucchini with the minty salsa.

Nutrition:

- Calories: 71
- Fat: 5 g
- Carbs: 6 g
- Protein: 2 g

Broccoli Cream

Preparation Time: 5 minutes
Cooking Time: 20 minutes
Servings: 4
Ingredients:
- 1 pound broccoli florets
- 4 cups vegetable stock
- 2 chopped shallots
- 1 teaspoon chili powder
- Salt
- Black pepper
- 2 minced garlic cloves
- 2 tablespoons olive oil
- 1 tablespoon chopped dill

Directions:
1. Heat up a pot with the oil over medium-high heat; add the shallots and the garlic and sauté for 2 minutes.
2. Add the broccoli and the other ingredients bring to a simmer, then cook over medium heat for 18 minutes.
3. Blend the mix using an immersion blender, divide the cream into bowls, and serve.

Nutrition:
- Calories: 111
- Fat: 8 g
- Carbs: 10.2 g
- Protein: 3.7 g

Linguine with Wild Mushrooms

Preparation Time: 5 minutes

Cooking Time: 10 minutes

Servings: 4

Ingredients:

- 12 ounces mixed mushrooms, sliced
- 2 green onions, sliced
- 1 1/2 teaspoon minced garlic
- 1 pound whole-grain linguine pasta,
- 1/4 cups nutritional yeast
- 1/2 teaspoon salt
- 3/4 teaspoon ground black pepper
- 6 tablespoons olive oil
- 3/4 cups vegetable stock, hot

Directions:

1. Take a skillet pan, place it over medium-high heat, add garlic and mushroom, and cook for 5 minutes until tender.
2. Transfer the vegetables to a pot; add the cooked pasta and the remaining ingredients, except for green onions.
3. Garnish with green onions and serve.

Nutrition:

- Calories: 430
- Fat: 15 g
- Carbs: 62 g
- Protein: 15 g

Leeks Cream

Preparation Time: 5 minutes

Cooking Time: 30 minutes

Servings: 4

Ingredients:
- 4 sliced leeks
- 4 cups vegetable stock
- 1 tablespoon olive oil
- 2 chopped shallots
- 1 tablespoon chopped rosemary
- Pinch of salt
- Black pepper
- 1 cup heavy cream
- 1 tablespoon chopped chives

Directions:
1. Heat up a pot with the oil over medium-high heat; add the shallots and the leeks and sauté for 5 minutes.
2. Add the stock and the other ingredients except for the chives. Bring to a simmer, then cook over medium heat for 25 minutes, stirring from time to time.
3. Blend the soup using an immersion blender, ladle it into bowls, sprinkle the chives on top, and serve.

Nutrition:
- Calories: 150
- Fat: 3 g
- Carbs: 2 g
- Protein: 6 g

Eggplant Parmesan

Preparation Time: 5 minutes
Cooking Time: 45 minutes
Servings: 8
Ingredients:

- Cooking spray
- 28 ounces crushed tomatoes
- 2 eggplants, sliced into rounds
- 1/4 cups red wine
- 1/2 Salt and pepper
- 1 teaspoon dried basil
- 2 tablespoons olive oil
- 1 teaspoon dried oregano
- 1 cup onion, chopped
- 1/2 cups parmesan cheese
- 2 cloves garlic, crushed and
- 1 cup mozzarella cheese
- 2 Basil leaves, chopped

Directions:

1. Preheat your oven to 400°F.
2. Merge the ingredients except for the cheese and basil. Spray your baking pan with oil. Simmer for 10 minutes.
3. Arrange the eggplant in the baking pan. Spread the sauce on a baking dish. Season with salt and pepper. Top with the eggplant slices. Roast for 20 minutes.
4. Sprinkle the mozzarella and parmesan on top.
5. Over medium heat, set a pan in place. Attach the oil and cook the onion for 4 minutes. Bake in the oven for 25 minutes.
6. Add in garlic and cook for 2 more minutes.

Nutrition:
- Calories: 192
- Fat: 9 g
- Carbs: 16 g
- Protein: 10 g

Peppers and Lentils Salad

Preparation Time: 10 minutes
Cooking Time: 0 minutes
Servings: 4
Ingredients:

- 14 ounces canned lentils, drained and rinsed
- 2 spring onions, chopped
- 1 red bell pepper, chopped
- 1 green bell pepper, chopped
- 1 tablespoon fresh lime juice
- 1/3 cup coriander, chopped
- 2 teaspoon balsamic vinegar

Directions:

1. In a salad bowl, combine the lentils with the onions, bell peppers, and the rest of the ingredients, toss and serve.

Nutrition:

- Calories: 200
- Fat: 2.45 g
- Fiber: 6.7 g
- Carbs: 10.5 g
- Protein: 5.6 g; Protein: 10 g

Corn and Tomato Salad

Preparation Time: 10 minutes

Cooking Time: 0 minutes

Servings: 4

Ingredients:
- 2 avocados, pitted, peeled, and cubed
- 1 pint mixed cherry tomatoes, halved
- 2 tablespoons avocado oil
- 1 tablespoon lime juice
- 1/2 teaspoon lime zest, grated
- A pinch of salt and black pepper
- 1/4 cup dill, chopped

Directions:
1. In a salad bowl, mix the avocados with the tomatoes and the rest of the ingredients, toss, and serve cold.

Nutrition:
- Calories: 188
- Fat: 7.3 g
- Fiber: 4.9 g
- Carbs: 6.4 g
- Protein: 6.5 g

Orange and Cucumber Salad

Preparation Time: 10 minutes

Cooking Time: 0 minutes

Servings: 4

Ingredients:

- 2 cucumbers, sliced
- 1 orange, peeled and cut into segments
- 1 cup cherry tomatoes, halved
- 1 small red onion, chopped
- 3 tablespoons olive oil
- 4 1/2 teaspoons balsamic vinegar
- Salt and black pepper to the taste
- 1 tablespoon lemon juice

Directions:

1. Merge the cucumbers with the orange and the rest of the ingredients, toss and serve cold.

Nutrition:

- Calories: 102
- Fat: 7.5 g
- Fiber: 3 g
- Carbs: 6.1 g; Protein: 3.4 g

Greek Potato and Corn Salad

Preparation Time: 10 minutes
Cooking Time: 20 minutes
Servings: 2

Ingredients:
- 2 medium potatoes, peeled and cubed
- 2 shallots, chopped
- 1 tablespoon olive oil
- 2 cups corn
- 1 tablespoon dill, chopped
- 1 tablespoon balsamic vinegar
- Salt and black pepper to the taste

Directions:
1. Transfer the potatoes to a pot, add water to cover, bring to a simmer over medium heat, cook for 20 minutes, drain, and transfer to a bowl.
2. Add the shallots and the other ingredients, toss, and serve cold.

Nutrition:
- Calories: 198
- Fat: 5.3 g
- Fiber: 6.5 g
- Carbs: 11.6 g
- Protein: 4.5 g

Mint Cabbage Salad

Preparation Time: 10 minutes

Cooking Time: 0 minutes

Servings: 4

Ingredients:
- 1 small red onion, chopped
- 1 tablespoon olive oil
- 2 tablespoons lemon juice
- 1 tablespoon lemon zest, grated
- Salt and black pepper to the taste
- 1 green cabbage head, shredded
- 1/2 cup mint, chopped
- 1/4 cup pistachios, chopped

Directions:
1. Merge the cabbage with the mint, pistachios, and the rest of the ingredients, toss and serve cold.

Nutrition:
- Calories: 101
- Fat: 4.1 g
- Fiber: 3.1 g
- Carbs: 4.5 g; Protein: 4.6 g

Minty Mix

Preparation Time: 10 minutes
Cooking Time: 0 minutes
Servings: 2

Ingredients:
- 1/2 cups walnuts, chopped
- 2 cups cauliflower florets, steamed
- 1 teaspoon ginger, grated
- 1 garlic clove, minced
- 1 tablespoon mint, chopped
- Juice of 1/2 lemon
- Salt and pepper

Directions:
1. Merge the cauliflower with the walnuts and the rest of the ingredients, toss and serve.

Nutrition:
- Calories: 199
- Fat: 5.6 g
- Fiber: 4.5 g
- Carbs: 8.4 g; Protein: 3.5 g

Leeks Salad

Preparation Time: 10 minutes

Cooking Time: 0 minutes

Servings: 4

Ingredients:
- 1 tablespoon olive oil
- 4 leeks, sliced
- 3 garlic cloves, grated
- Salt and white pepper
- 1/2 teaspoon apple cider vinegar
- A drizzle of olive oil
- 1 tablespoon dill, chopped

Directions:
1. In a salad bowl, combine the leeks with the garlic and the rest of the ingredients, toss, and serve cold.

Nutrition:
- Calories: 71
- Fat: 2.1 g
- Fiber: 1.1 g
- Carbs: 1.3 g
- Protein: 2.4 g

Snow Peas Salad

Preparation Time: 6 hours
Cooking Time: 10 minutes
Servings: 4
Ingredients:

- 3 cups snow peas, trimmed
- 1 1/4 cup bean sprouts
- 1 tablespoon basil, chopped
- 1 tablespoon lime juice
- 1 teaspoon ginger, grated
- 2 spring onions, chopped
- 2 garlic cloves, minced

Directions:

1. Put the snow peas in a pot, add water to cover, bring to a simmer, and cook over medium heat for 10 minutes.
2. Drain the peas, transfer them to a bowl, add the sprouts, and the rest of the ingredients, toss and keep in the fridge for 6 hours before serving.

Nutrition:

- Calories: 200
- Fat: 8.6 g
- Fiber: 3 g
- Carbs: 5.4 g
- Protein: 3.4 g

Fennel and Zucchini Mix

Preparation Time: 10 minutes
Cooking Time: 15 minutes
Servings: 4
Ingredients:
- 1 cup fennel bulb, chopped
- 1 sweet onion, chopped
- 1 tablespoon olive oil
- 3 garlic cloves, minced
- 5 cups zucchini, roughly cubed
- 1 cup veggie stock
- Salt and black pepper the taste
- 2 teaspoons white wine vinegar
- 1 teaspoon lemon juice

Directions:
1. Heat the oil and add the onion and the garlic, toss, and sauté for 5 minutes.
2. Merge the rest of the ingredients, toss, cook for 10 minutes more, divide into bowls, and serve.

Nutrition:
- Calories: 193
- Fat: 3 g
- Fiber: 2.4 g
- Carbs: 3 g
- Protein: 2.3 g

Orange Potato Salad

Preparation Time: 10 minutes
Cooking Time: 40 minutes
Servings: 4
Ingredients:

- 4 sweet potatoes
- 3 tablespoons olive oil
- 1/3 cup orange juice
- 1/2 teaspoon sumac, ground
- 1 tablespoon red wine vinegar
- Salt and black pepper to the taste
- 1 tablespoon orange zest, grated
- 2 tablespoons mint, chopped
- 1/3 cup walnuts, chopped
- 1/3 cup pomegranate seeds

Directions:

1. Put the potatoes on a lined baking sheet, introduce them in the oven at 350°F bake for 40 minutes, cool them down, peel, cut into wedges, and transfer to a bowl.
2. Merge the rest of the ingredients, toss, and serve cold.

Nutrition:

- Calories: 138
- Fat: 3.5 g
- Fiber: 6.2 g
- Carbs: 10.4 g
- Protein: 6.5 g

Avocado Sticks

Preparation Time: 5 minutes
Cooking Time: 10 minutes
Servings: 2
Ingredients:
- 2 avocados
- 1 c. coconut flour
- 2 tsps. black pepper
- 3 egg yolks
- 1½ tbsps. water
- ¼ tsp. salt
- 1 c. vegan butter
- 2 tsps. minced garlic
- ¼ c. chopped parsley
- 1 tbsp. lemon juice

Directions:
1. Place butter in a mixing bowl then adds minced garlic, chopped parsley, and lemon juice to the bowl.
2. Using an electric mixer mix until smooth and fluffy.
3. Transfer the garlic butter to a container with a lid then store in the fridge.
4. Peel the avocados then cut into wedges. Set aside.
5. Put the egg yolks in a mixing bowl then pour water into it.
6. Season with salt and black pepper, then stir until incorporated.
7. Take an avocado wedge then roll in the coconut flour.
8. Dip in the egg mixture then returns back to the coconut flour. Roll until the avocado wedge is completely coated. Repeat with the remaining avocado wedges.
9. Preheat an Air Fryer to 400°F (204°C).

10. Arrange the coated avocado wedges in the Air Fryer basket then cook for 8 minutes or until golden.
11. Remove from the Air Fryer then arrange on a serving dish.
12. Serve with garlic butter then enjoy right away.

Nutrition:

- Calories: 340,
- Fat: 33.8g,
- Protein: 4.5g,
- Carbs: 8.5g 148

Sizzling Vegetarian Fajitas

Preparation Time: 5 minutes
Cooking Time: 120 minutes
Servings: 2
Ingredients:

- 4 oz. diced green chilies
- ½ tsp. garlic powder
- 3 diced tomatoes
- ¼ tsp. salt
- 1 cored yellow bell pepper,
- 2 tsps. red chili powder
- sliced
- 2 tsps. ground cumin
- 1 cored red bell pepper,
- ½ tsp. dried oregano
- sliced
- 1 ½ tbsps. olive oil
- 1 white onion, peeled and
- sliced

Directions:

1. Take a 6-quarts slow cooker, grease it Plug in the slow cooker; adjust the
2. with a non-stick cooking spray, and
3. cooking time to 2 hours and let it
4. add all the ingredients.
5. cook on the high heat setting or until cooks thoroughly.
6. Stir until it mixes properly and cover STEP 4
7. the top.
8. Serve with tortilla.

Nutrition:

- Calories: 220
- Cal, Carbs: 73g,
- Protein: 12g,
- Fats: 8g 151

Spinach and Feta Pita Bake

Preparation Time: 5 minutes
Cooking Time: 12 minutes
Servings: 3
Ingredients:

- 6 oz. tomato pesto
- 6 whole wheat pita breads
- 2 chopped tomatoes
- ½ c. Kalamata olives
- mushrooms, feta cheese.
- 1 bunch chopped spinach
- 4 sliced mushrooms
- ½ c. crumbled feta cheese
- pepper for seasoning.
- 3 tbsps. olive oil

Directions:

1. Set oven to 350 degrees F.
2. Spread tomato pesto onto one side of each pita bread and place them pesto-side up on a baking sheet.
3. Top pitas with spinach, tomatoes,
4. Sprinkle with olive oil, and add
5. Bake in preheated oven 10-12 minutes or until pitas are crisp. Cut into quarters and serve.

Nutrition:
350 Calories, 11g Protein, 17g Fat, 41g Carbs 152

Quinoa And Spinach Cakes

Preparation Time: 5 minutes
Cooking Time: 9 minutes
Servings: 2
Ingredients:

- 2 c. cooked quinoa
- 1 c. chopped baby spinach
- 1 egg
- 2 tbsps. minced parsley
- 1 tsp. minced garlic
- 1 carrot, peeled and shredded
- 1 chopped onion
- ¼ c. oat milk
- ¼ c. parmesan cheese, grated
- 1 c. breadcrumbs
- sea salt
- ground black peppe

Directions:

1. In a mixing bowl, mix all ingredients.
2. Season with salt and pepper to taste.
3. Preheat your Air Fryer to 390°F.
4. Scoop ¼ cup of quinoa and spinach mixture and place in the Air Fryer cooking basket. Cook in batches until browned for about 8 minutes.
5. Serve and enjoy!

Nutrition:

- Calories: 188
- Fat: 4.4 g
- Carbs: 31.2g; Protein: 8.1g 157

Garlicky Kale & Pea Saute

Preparation Time: 5 minutes

Cooking Time: 8 minutes

Servings: 2

Ingredients:

- 2 sliced garlic cloves
- 1 chopped hot red chile
- 2 tbsps. olive oil
- 2 bunches chopped kale
- 1 lb. frozen peas

Directions:

1. In a saucepot, mix the ingredients except peas. Cook until the kale becomes tender for about 6 minutes.
2. Add peas and cook for 2 more minutes.

Nutrition:

85 Calories, 3g Fats, 11g Net Carbs, and 5g Protein 158

Mashed Cauliflower

Preparation Time: 5 minutes
Cooking Time: 6 minutes
Servings: 4
Ingredients:

- 1 head cauliflower head
- 3 tbsps. melt vegetarian butter
- 1 c. water
- ¼ c. pepper
- ½ tsp. salt

Directions:

1. Chop the cauliflower and place inside the steamer basket.
2. Pour the water into the Instant Pot and lower the basket.
3. Close the lid, set it to MANUAL, and cook at high pressure for 4 minutes.
4. Do a quick pressure release.
5. Mash the cauliflower with a potato masher or in a food processor and stir in the remaining ingredients.
6. Serve and enjoy!

Nutrition:

- Calories: 113
- Fat: 5.9 g
- Carbs: 4.1 g
- Protein: 3 g 161

Sun-dried Tomato Pesto

Preparation Time: 5 minutes

Cooking Time: 11 minutes

Servings: 5

Ingredients:

- 1 c. fresh basil leaves
- 6 oz. sun-dried tomatoes
- 1 tbsp. lemon juice
- ½ tsp. salt
- ¼ c. olive oil
- ¼ c. almonds
- 3 minced garlic cloves
- ½ tsp. chopped red pepper
- 8 oz. pasta

Directions:

1. Cook the pasta according to the given instructions. For making, the pesto, toasts the almonds over medium flame in a small skillet for around 4 minutes.
2. In a blender, put sun-dried tomatoes, basil, garlic, lemon juice, salt, red pepper flakes, and toasted almonds and blend it. While blending adds olive oil in it and blend it until it converts in the form of a pesto. flakes
3. Now coat the pasta with the pesto and serve it.

Nutrition:

- Calories 256,
- Fat 13.7g,
- Carbs 28.1g,
- Protein 6.7g 16

Grilled Zuchinni

Preparation Time: 5 minutes
Cooking Time: 10 minutes
Servings: 2
Ingredients:

- 4 zucchinis, sliced
- 1 tbsp. olive oil
- salt and pepper
- 1 c. tomatoes, chopped
- 1 tbsp. mint, chopped
- 1 tsp. red wine vinegar

Directions:

1. Preheat your grill.
2. Coat the zucchini with oil and season with salt and pepper.
3. Grill for 4 minutes per side.
4. Mix the remaining ingredients in a bowl.
5. Top the grilled zucchini with the minty salsa.

Nutrition:

- Calories 71,
- Fat 5 g,
- Carbs 6 g,
- Protein 2 g 170

Eggplant Italiano

Preparation Time: 5 minutes
Cooking Time: 5 minutes
Servings: 8
Ingredients:

- 2½ lbs. eggplant, cubed
- 4 celery stalks, cut into 1-inch
- 2 sliced onions
- 7½ oz. canned tomato sauce
- 2 cans (16 ounce each) diced
- 2 tbsps. olive oil, divided
- 1 c. olives pitted and halved
- 4 tbsps. balsamic vinegar
- 2 tbsps. drained capers
- 1 tbsp. maple syrup
- 2 tsps. dried basil
- salt
- pepper
- basil leaves to garnish

Directions:

1. Add all the ingredients into the
2. Instant Pot. Stir to mix well
3. Close the lid. Select MANUAL and cook at high pressure for 4 minutes.
4. When the cooking is complete, do a quick pressure release.
5. Garnish with fresh basil and serve over rice or noodles.

Nutrition:

- Calories: 127; Fat: 5.8 g; Carbs: 11.6 ; Protein: 3 g 174

Balsamic-Glazed Roasted

Preparation Time: 5 minutes
Cooking Time: 75 minutes
Servings: 4
Ingredients:
- 1 head cauliflower
- ½ lb. green beans, trimmed
- 1 peeled red onion, wedged
- 2 c. cherry tomatoes
- ½ tsp. salt
- ¼ c. brown sugar
- 3 tbsps. olive oil
- 1 c. balsamic vinegar
- 2 tbsps. chopped parsley, for

Directions:
1. Place cauliflower florets in a baking dish, add tomatoes, green beans, and onion wedges around it, season with salt, and drizzle with oil.
2. Pour vinegar in a saucepan, stir in sugar, bring the mixture to a boil and simmer for 15 minutes until reduced by half.
3. Brush the sauce generously over cauliflower florets and then roast for 1 hour at 400 degrees f until cooked, brushing sauce frequently.
4. When done, garnish vegetables with parsley and then serve.

Nutrition:

- Calories: 86
- Fat: 5.7 g
- Carbs: 7.7 g; Protein: 3.1 g 177

Charred Green Beans with Mustard

Preparation Time: 5 minutes

Cooking Time: 20 minutes

Servings: 2

Ingredients:

- 1 teaspoon whole-grain mustard
- 1/8 teaspoon salt
- 1/8 teaspoon black pepper
- 1½ tablespoons olive oil, divided
- ½ pound green beans, trimmed
- ½ tablespoon red-wine vinegar
- 1/8 cup toasted hazelnuts, chopped

Directions:

1. Preheat a grill on high heat and grease a grill pan.
2. Mix green beans with ½ tablespoon of olive oil in a pan.
3. Transfer to the grill pan and grill the beans for about 8 minutes.
4. Mix the beans with mustard, olive oil, vinegar, salt and black pepper.
5. Top with hazelnuts and serve hot.

Nutrition:

- Calories 181
- Total Fat 14.6 g
- Saturated Fat 2.3 g
- Cholesterol 97 mg
- Total Carbs 8.5 g
- Dietary Fiber 6.1 g
- Sugar 2.4 g
- Protein 2.8 g

Lemony Mushroom and Herb Rice

Preparation Time: 5 minutes

Cooking Time: 20 minutes

Servings: 8

Ingredients:
- 4 large garlic cloves, finely chopped
- ¼ cup parsley, chopped
- 6 tablespoons chives, snipped
- 2½ cups chestnut mushrooms, diced
- 2 cups long grain rice
- 4 tablespoons olive oil
- 2 lemons, zested

Direction:
1. Boil water with salt in a pan and add rice.
2. Cook for about 10 minutes while stirring continuously and drain them through a sieve.
3. Sauté mushrooms for about 5 minutes and stir in the garlic cloves.
4. Sauté for about 1 minute and toss in chives, parsley, lemon zest and drained rice.
5. Dish out to serve and enjoy.

Nutrition:
- Calories 281
- Total Fat 8.9 g
- Saturated Fat 1.4 g
- Cholesterol 0 mg
- Total Carbs 43.6 g
- Dietary Fiber 5.4 g ; Sugar 0.8 g ; Protein 9 g

Smoky Roasted Vegetables

Preparation Time: 10 minutes

Cooking Time: 1 hour 40 minutes

Servings: 4

Ingredients:

- ½ orange bell pepper, sliced
- 1 bay leaf
- 1 small red onion, sliced into rounds and separated
- ½ summer squash, cut into 3-inch sticks
- ½ teaspoon sea salt, divided
- 1/6 cup extra-virgin olive oil
- 2 small tomatoes, sliced
- ½ yellow bell pepper, sliced
- ½ zucchini, cut into 3-inch sticks
- 1 sprig fresh thyme
- ½ tablespoon balsamic vinegar
- ½ tablespoon red-wine vinegar
- ½ eggplant, cut into 3-inch sticks
- 2 sprigs fresh parsley
- 2 garlic cloves, divided

Direction:

1. Preheat the oven to 360 degrees F and lightly grease a baking dish.
2. Season all the vegetables with salt and transfer to the baking dish.
3. Tie parsley, thyme and bay leaf with a kitchen string and place them at the center of the seasoned vegetables.
4. Drizzle with oil and top with garlic cloves.
5. Transfer in the oven and bake for about 1 hour 15 minutes.

6. Drizzle with vinegar and serve immediately.

Nutrition:

- Calories 231
- Total Fat 17.5 g
- Saturated Fat 2.5 g
- Cholesterol 0 mg
- Total Carbs 19.6 g
- Dietary Fiber 7.3 g
- Sugar 10.6 g
- Protein 3.6 g

Cashew and Bell Pepper Rice

Preparation Time: 5 minutes

Cooking Time: 15minutes

Servings: 2

Ingredients:

- 2 oz. cashew nuts
- ½ yellow bell pepper, deseeded and finely sliced
- 1½ cups cooked basmati rice, cooled
- ½ green bell pepper, deseeded and finely sliced
- ½ small red onion, finely sliced
- For the dressing
- ½ tablespoon brown sugar
- 1 tablespoon light soy sauce
- ¼ lemon, juiced
- 1½ tablespoons mango chutney
- 1 teaspoon curry powder
- ½ tablespoon oil

Directions:

1. Mix together all the ingredients for dressing in a bowl.
2. Toast the cashews until golden brown and transfer to the mixed dressing.
3. Toss in rice, onions and bell peppers and immediately serve.

Nutrition:

- Calories 433
- Total Fat 17.1 g
- Saturated Fat 3.2 g
- Cholesterol 0 mg
- Total Carbs 70.6 g
- Dietary Fiber 2.5 g ; Sugar 14.1 g ; Protein 10.3 g

Roasted Vegetable Tabbouleh

Preparation Time: 5 minutes

Cooking Time: 35 minutes

Servings: 2

Ingredients:

- 1 (8-ounce) can garbanzo beans, rinsed and drained
- ¼ cup fresh parsley, chopped
- 2 small carrots, chopped
- 1/3 cup bulgur, boiled and drained
- ½ small red onion, chopped
- 1½ tablespoons lemon juice
- ¼ teaspoon black pepper
- ¼ teaspoon lemon peel, finely shredded
- 1 tablespoon water
- ½ medium tomatoes, chopped
- 1 tablespoon olive oil
- 1/8 teaspoon salt
- 1 teaspoon fresh thyme, snipped

Directions:

1. Preheat the oven to 390 degrees F and lightly grease a baking dish.
2. Organize carrots and onions in a baking dish and drizzle with olive oil.
3. Bake for about 25 minutes and dish out in a bowl.
4. Add lemon peel, pepper, salt, bulgur, parsley, lemon juice and garbanzo to the baked veggies bowl and immediately serve.

Nutrition:

- Calories 370
- Total Fat 10.6 g
- Saturated Fat 1.5 g
- Cholesterol 0 mg
- Total Carbs 58.7 g
- Dietary Fiber 15.9 g
- Sugar 9.6 g
- Protein 14.1 g

Moroccan Couscous

Preparation Time: 5 minutes
Cooking Time: 20 minutes
Servings: 16
Ingredients:

- 2/3 cup dried apricots, chopped
- 2 oranges, juiced
- 2/3 cup golden raisins
- 1 teaspoon ground ginger
- 2 oranges, zested
- ½ teaspoon ground cinnamon
- 3 cups vegetable stock
- 2/3 cup dates, chopped
- 1 teaspoon ground cumin
- 4 cups whole-wheat couscous
- 1 cup slivered almonds, toasted
- ½ teaspoon coriander
- 2 tablespoons butter
- Salt, to taste
- 1 teaspoon turmeric
- ½ cup mint, chopped

Directions:

1. Boil stock in a saucepan and add orange juice, zest, dates, apricots, raisins, couscous and spices.
2. Remove the pan from heat and allow the couscous to absorb the liquid for about 15 minutes.
3. Stir in the butter, mint and almonds and sprinkle with salt to serve.

Nutrition:

- Calories 264
- Total Fat 5 g
- Saturated Fat 1 g
- Cholesterol 4 mg
- Total Carbs 48 g
- Dietary Fiber 4 g
- Sugar 7.5 g
- Protein 8 g

Parmesan Roasted Broccoli

Preparation Time: 5 minutes
Cooking Time: 35 minutes
Servings: 8
Ingredients:
- 1 cup Parmesan cheese, grated
- 2 pounds broccoli florets, cut into bite-sized pieces
- 4 tablespoons olive oil
- 2 lemons, zested
- ¼ teaspoon sea salt
- Salt, to taste
- ¼ teaspoon red pepper flakes
- 4 tablespoons balsamic vinegar

Directions:
1. Preheat the oven to 395 degrees F and lightly grease a baking sheet.
2. Season the broccoli florets with salt and place on the baking sheet.
3. Bake for about 15 minutes and top with parmesan cheese.
4. Bake these florets again for about 10 minutes and dish out in a bowl.
5. Season with lemon zest, salt, red pepper flakes and balsamic vinegar to serve.

Nutrition:
- Calories 146
- Total Fat 10.4 g
- Saturated Fat 3 g ; Cholesterol 10 mg
- Total Carbs 8.5 g ; Dietary Fiber 3 g
- Sugar 2.4 g ; Protein 7.7 g

Spinach Beans

Preparation Time: 10 minutes
Cooking Time: 30 minutes
Servings: 4
Ingredients:

- 2 cans (14½ ounces) diced tomatoes, undrained
- 2 cans (15 ounces) cannellini beans, rinsed and drained
- 4 garlic cloves, minced
- ½ teaspoon black pepper
- 28 ounces bacon, chopped
- 2 small onions, chopped
- ½ teaspoon salt
- 12 ounces fresh baby spinach
- 2 tablespoons olive oil
- 4 tablespoons Worcestershire sauce
- ¼ teaspoon red pepper flakes, crushed

Directions:

1. Heat oil in a skillet on medium heat and add bacon.
2. Sauté until brown and stir in the garlic and onions.
3. Sauté for about 5 minutes and add Worcestershire sauce, seasonings and tomatoes.
4. Reduce the heat and cook for about 10 minutes.
5. Toss in the beans and spinach and cook for about 5 minutes.
6. Stir well and serve immediately.

Nutrition:

- Calories 475 ; Total Fat 8.5 g
- Saturated Fat 1.2 g ; Cholesterol 0 mg
- Total Carbs 77.8 g ; Dietary Fiber 31.1 g
- Sugar 10.1 g ; Protein 28.2 g

Roasted Carrots Recipe

Preparation Time: 5 min

Cooking Time: 30 min

Servings: 6

Ingredient:

- ½ tablespoon of a lime juice
- ½ teaspoon of ground turmeric
- Kosher Salt
- 1 finely minced garlic clove
- Black pepper
- Extra virgin olive oil
- 2 lb. peeled carrots
- Parsley

Directions:

1. Preheat the oven at 400 degrees F and get a large mixing bowl. Pour the sliced carrots in it and spray it with extra virgin olive oil. Stir to ensure that the oil circulates to the carrots, then spice it with salt and pepper. Arrange the carrots into a baking sheet and cook for about 20 min. turn them at about half time to ensure that the color remains balanced on both sides. Then take it out of the oven and serve. Here is the time to season with your turmeric and garnish with fresh parsley.

Nutrition:

- 67.5 kcal
- 0.7g of fat
- 4.6g of fiber ; 0.7mg of iron
- 51.4mg of calcium ; 13.2g of carbs ; 1.98g of protein.

Homemade Pita Chips

Preparation Time: 5 min
Cooking Time: 10 min
Servings: 6
Ingredient:
- 2 pita breads that have pockets
- Kosher salt
- Extra virgin olive oil
- Use any seasoning.

Directions:
1. Preheat the oven at 430 degrees F and get a large baking sheet near. Get a large cutting board and place each pita on it. Use kitchen shears to cut them into halves, you can equally use a knife. I advise you should not use the thick single layered pitas so that you can easily follow this step. If that's what you are using, however, do not bother to cut it into halves. Stroke all sides of the pita with the extra virgin olive oil and add your salt to it. Brush it with your seasoning too. Take each pita and cut into 8 triangles and place them in the baking sheet. Bake for about 7 min and turn it over once in a while to ensure that the colors on the two sides are balanced.

Nutrition:
- 14.4 kcal
- 0.3g of fat
- 27mg of sodium
- 5mg of calcium
- 0.3mg of Iron
- 2.8g of carbs ; 0.5g of protein.

Chapter 2. Salad

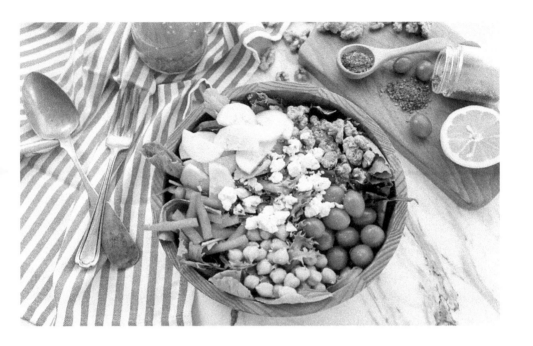

Lentil Salmon Salad

Preparation Time: 25 minutes

Cooking Time: 25 minutes

Servings: 4

Ingredients:

- 2 cups vegetable stock
- 1 rinsed green lentils
- 1 chopped red onion
- 1/2 cup chopped parsley
- 4 ounces shredded smoked salmon
- 2 tablespoons chopped cilantro
- 1 chopped red pepper
- 1 lemon, juiced
- Salt and pepper to taste

Directions:

1. Cook vegetable stock and lentils in a saucepan for 15 to 20 minutes, on low heat. Ensure all liquid has been absorbed and then remove from heat.
2. Pour into a salad bowl and top with red pepper, parsley, cilantro, and salt and pepper (to suit your taste) and mix.
3. Mix in lemon juice and shredded salmon.
4. This salad should be served fresh.

Nutrition:

- Calories: 260
- Fat: 2 g
- Fiber: 8 g
- Carbs: 17 g
- Protein: 11 g

Peppy Pepper Tomato Salad

Preparation Time: 20 minutes

Cooking Time: 20 minutes

Servings: 4

Ingredients:

- 1 yellow bell pepper, cored and diced
- 4 cucumbers, diced
- 1 red onion, chopped
- 1 tablespoon balsamic vinegar
- 2 tablespoons extra-virgin olive oil
- 4 diced tomatoes
- 2 cored and diced red bell peppers
- 1 pinch chili flakes
- Salt and pepper to taste

Directions:

1. Merge all above ingredients in a salad bowl, except salt and pepper.
2. Season with salt and pepper to suit your taste and mix well.
3. Eat while fresh.

Nutrition:

- Calories: 260
- Fat: 2 g
- Fiber: 8 g
- Carbs: 17 g
- Protein: 11 g

Bulgur Salad

Preparation Time: 20 minutes

Cooking Time: 30 minutes

Servings: 4

Ingredients:

- 2 cups vegetable stock
- 2/3 cup uncooked bulgur
- 1 garlic clove, minced
- 1 cup cherry tomatoes, halved
- 2 tablespoons Almonds, sliced
- 1/4 cup, pitted and chopped
- 1 tablespoon lemon juice
- 8 ounces baby spinach
- 1 cucumber, diced
- 1 tablespoon balsamic vinegar
- Salt and pepper to taste
- 2 tablespoons mixed seeds

Directions:

1. Pour the stock into saucepan and heat until hot, and then stir in bulgur and cook until the bulgur has absorbed all stock.
2. Put in a salad bowl and add the remaining ingredients, stir well.
3. Season salt and pepper to suit your taste.
4. Serve and eat immediately.

Nutrition:

- Calories: 260
- Fat: 2 g
- Fiber: 8 g
- Carbs: 17 g
- Protein: 11 g

Tasty Tuna Salad

Preparation Time: 15 minutes

Cooking Time: 30 minutes

Servings: 4

Ingredients:

- 1/4 cup, sliced green olives
- 1 can, drained tuna in water
- 2 tablespoons pine nuts
- 1 jar artichoke hearts, drained and chopped
- 2 tablespoons extra-virgin olive oil
- 1, juiced lemon
- 2 leaves arugula
- 1 tablespoon Dijon mustard
- Salt and pepper to taste

Directions:

1. Merge mustard, oil, and lemon juice in a bowl to make a dressing. Combine the artichoke hearts, tuna, green olives, arugula, and pine nuts in a salad bowl.
2. In a separate salad bowl, mix tuna, arugula, pine nuts, artichoke hearts, and tuna.
3. Pour dressing mix onto the salad and serve fresh.

Nutrition:

- Calories: 260
- Fat: 3 g
- Fiber: 10 g
- Carbs: 20 g
- Protein: 9 g

Sweet and Sour Spinach Salad

Preparation Time: 15 minutes

Cooking Time: 30 minutes

Servings: 4

Ingredients:
- 2 sliced red onions
- 4 baby spinach leaves
- 1/2 teaspoon sesame oil
- 2 tablespoons apple cider vinegar
- 1 teaspoon honey
- 2 tablespoons sesame seeds
- Salt and pepper to taste

Directions:
1. Mix together honey, sesame oil, vinegar, and sesame seeds in a small bowl to make a dressing. Attach in salt and pepper to suit your taste.
2. Attach red onions and spinach together in a salad bowl.
3. Pour dressing over the salad and serve while cool and fresh.

Nutrition:
- Calories: 260
- Fat: 3 g
- Fiber: 10 g
- Carbs: 20 g
- Protein: 9 g

Easy Eggplant Salad

Preparation Time: 15 minutes

Cooking Time: 30 minutes

Servings: 4

Ingredients:
- Salt and pepper to taste
- 2 eggplant, sliced
- 1 teaspoon smoked paprika
- 2 tablespoons extra-virgin olive oil
- 2 garlic cloves, minced
- 2 cups mixed greens
- 2 tablespoons sherry vinegar

Directions:
1. Mix together garlic, paprika, and oil in a small bowl.
2. Place eggplant on a plate and sprinkle with salt and pepper to suit your taste. Next, brush the oil mixture onto the eggplant.
3. Cook eggplant on a medium heated grill pan until brown on both sides. Once cooked, put eggplant into a salad bowl.
4. Top with greens and vinegar, serve, and eat.

Nutrition:
- Calories: 110
- Fat: 3.5 g
- Fiber: 10.3 g
- Carbs: 18 g
- Protein: 9 g

Sweetest Sweet Potato Salad

Preparation Time: 15 minutes

Cooking Time: 30 minutes

Servings: 4

Ingredients:

- 2 tablespoons honey
- 1 teaspoon sumac spice
- 2 finely sliced sweet potato
- 3 tablespoons extra-virgin olive oil
- 1 teaspoon dried mint
- 1 tablespoon balsamic vinegar
- Salt and pepper to taste
- 1 seeded pomegranate
- 3 cups mixed greens

Directions:

1. Place sweet potato slices on a plate and add sumac, mint, salt, and pepper on both sides. Next, drizzle oil and honey over both sides.
2. Attach oil to a grill pan and heat. Grill sweet potatoes on medium heat until brown on both sides.
3. Put sweet potatoes in a salad bowl and top with pomegranate and mixed greens.
4. Stir and eat right away.

Nutrition:

- Calories: 110
- Fat: 3.5 g
- Fiber: 10.3 g
- Carbs: 18 g
- Protein: 9 g

Delicious Chickpea Salad

Preparation Time: 15 minutes

Cooking Time: 30 minutes

Servings: 4

Ingredients:

- 1 can chickpeas, drained
- 1 cup cherry tomatoes, quartered
- 1/2 cup parsley, chopped
- 1/2 cup red seedless grapes, halved
- 4 ounces feta cheese, cubed
- Salt and pepper to taste
- 1 tablespoon lemon juice
- 1/4 cup Greek yogurt
- 2 tablespoons extra-virgin olive oil

Directions:

1. In a salad bowl, mix together parsley, chickpeas, grapes, feta cheese, and tomatoes.
2. Add in the remaining ingredients, seasoning with salt and pepper to suit your taste.
3. This fresh salad is best when served right away.

Nutrition:

- Calories: 115
- Fat: 4 g
- Fiber: 11 g
- Carbs: 20 g
- Protein: 10 g

Couscous Arugula Salad

Preparation Time: 15 minutes

Cooking Time: 20 minutes

Servings: 4

Ingredients:

- 1/2 cup couscous
- 1 cup vegetable stock
- 1 bunch, peeled asparagus
- 1 lemon, juiced
- 1 teaspoon dried tarragon
- 2 cups arugula
- Salt and pepper to taste

Directions:

1. Heat the vegetable stock in a pot until hot. Remove from heat and add in the couscous. Cover until the couscous has absorbed all the stock.
2. Pour in a bowl and fluff with a fork and then set aside to cool.
3. Peel asparagus with a vegetable peeler, making them into ribbons and put into a bowl with couscous.
4. Merge the remaining ingredients and add salt and pepper to suit your taste.
5. Serve the salad immediately.

Nutrition:

- Calories: 100
- Fat: 6 g
- Fiber: 13 g
- Carbs: 25 g
- Protein: 10 g

Spinach and Grilled Feta Salad

Preparation Time: 10 minutes

Cooking Time: 25 minutes

Servings: 4

Ingredients:

- 8 ounces feta cheese, sliced
- 1/4 cup black olives, sliced
- 1/4 cup green olives, sliced
- 4 cups baby spinach
- 2 garlic cloves, minced
- 1 teaspoon capers, chopped
- 2 tablespoons extra-virgin olive oil
- 1 tablespoon red wine vinegar

Directions:

1. Grill feta cheese slices over medium to high flame until brown on both sides.
2. In a salad bowl, mix green olives, black olives, and spinach.
3. In a separate bowl, mix vinegar, capers, and oil together to make a dressing.
4. Top salad with the dressing and cheese, and it is ready to serve.

Nutrition:

- Calories: 100
- Fat: 6 g
- Fiber: 13 g
- Carbs: 25 g
- Protein: 10 g

Creamy Cool Salad

Preparation Time: 10 minutes

Cooking Time: 25 minutes

Servings: 4

Ingredients:

- 1/2 cup Greek yogurt
- 2 tablespoons dill, chopped
- 1 teaspoon lemon juice
- 4 cucumbers, diced
- 2 garlic cloves, minced
- Salt and pepper to taste

Directions:

1. Mix all ingredients in a salad bowl.
2. Season with salt and pepper to suit your taste and eat.

Nutrition:

- Calories: 115
- Fat: 9 g
- Fiber: 10 g
- Carbs: 21 g
- Protein: 9 g

Grilled Salmon Summer Salad

Preparation Time: 10 minutes

Cooking Time: 30 minutes

Servings: 4

Ingredients:
- 2 salmon fillets
- Salt and pepper to taste
- 2 cups vegetable stock
- 1/2 cup bulgur
- 1 cup cherry tomatoes, halved
- 1/2 cup sweet corn
- 1 lemon, juiced
- 1/2 cup green olives, sliced
- 1 cucumber, cubed
- 1 green onion, chopped
- 1 red pepper, chopped
- 1 red bell pepper, cored and diced

Directions:
1. Heat a grill pan on medium and then place salmon on, seasoning with salt and pepper. Grill both sides of the salmon until brown and set aside.
2. Heat stock in a saucepan until hot and then add in bulgur and cook until liquid is completely soaked into bulgur.
3. Mix salmon, bulgur, and all other ingredients in a salad bowl, and again add salt and pepper, if desired, to suit your taste.
4. Serve the salad as soon as completed.

Nutrition:
- Calories: 110; Fat: 13 g
- Fiber: 7 g; Carbs: 13 g; Protein: 18 g

Broccoli Salad with Caramelized Onions

Preparation Time: 10 minutes

Cooking Time: 25 minutes

Servings: 4

Ingredients:
- 3 tablespoons extra-virgin olive oil
- 2 red onions, sliced
- 1 teaspoon dried thyme
- 2 tablespoons balsamic vinegar
- 1 pound broccoli, cut into florets
- Salt and pepper to taste

Directions:
1. Heat the oil and add in sliced onions. Cook until the onions are caramelized. Stir in vinegar and thyme and then remove from the stove.
2. Mix together the broccoli and onion mixture in a bowl, adding salt and pepper if desired. Serve and eat salad as soon as possible.

Nutrition:
- Calories: 113
- Fat: 9 g
- Fiber: 8 g
- Carbs: 13 g
- Protein: 18 g

Baked Cauliflower Mixed Salad

Preparation Time: 10 minutes

Cooking Time: 30 minutes

Servings: 4

Ingredients:
- 2 tablespoons extra-virgin olive oil
- 1 teaspoon dried mint
- 1 teaspoon dried oregano
- 2 tablespoons chopped parsley
- 1 red pepper, chopped
- 1 lemon, juiced
- 1 green onion, chopped
- 2 tablespoons chopped cilantro
- Salt and pepper to taste

Directions:
1. Heat oven to 350°F.
2. In a deep baking pan, combine olive oil, mint, cauliflower, and oregano, and bake for 15 minutes.
3. Once cooked, pour into a salad bowl, and add the remaining ingredients, stirring together.
4. Plate the salad and eat fresh and warm.

Nutrition:
- Calories: 123
- Fat: 13 g
- Fiber: 9 g
- Carbs: 10 g
- Protein: 12.5 g

Quick Arugula Salad

Preparation Time: 10 minutes

Cooking Time: 30 minutes

Servings: 4

Ingredients:

- 6 roasted red bell peppers, sliced
- 2 tablespoons pine nuts
- 2 tablespoons dried raisins
- 1 red onion, sliced
- 3 cups arugula
- 2 tablespoons balsamic vinegar
- 4 ounces feta cheese, crumbled
- 2 tablespoons extra-virgin olive oil
- 4 ounces feta cheese, crumbled
- Salt and pepper to taste

Directions:

1. Using a salad bowl, combine vinegar, olive oil, pine nuts, raisins, peppers, and onions.
2. Add arugula and feta cheese to the mix and serve.

Nutrition:

- Calories: 123
- Fat: 13 g
- Fiber: 9 g
- Carbs: 10 g
- Protein: 12 g

Bell Pepper and Tomato Salad

Preparation Time: 10 minutes

Cooking Time: 15 minutes

Servings: 4

Ingredients:

- 8 roasted red bell pepper, sliced
- 2 tablespoons extra-virgin olive oil
- 1 pinch chili flakes
- 4 garlic cloves, minced
- 2 tablespoons pine nuts
- 1 shallot, sliced
- 1 cup cherry tomatoes, halved
- 2 tablespoons parsley, chopped
- 1 tablespoon balsamic vinegar
- Salt and pepper to taste

Directions:

1. Merge all ingredients except salt and pepper in a salad bowl.
2. Season with salt and pepper if you want, to suit your taste.
3. Eat once freshly made.

Nutrition:

- Calories: 112
- Fat: 11 g
- Fiber: 8 g
- Carbs: 10 g
- Protein: 12 g

One Bowl Spinach Salad

Preparation Time: 10 minutes

Cooking Time: 20 minutes

Servings: 4

Ingredients:
- 2 red beets, cooked and diced
- 1 tablespoon apple cider vinegar
- 3 cups baby spinach
- 1/4 cup Greek yogurt
- 1 tablespoon horseradish
- Salt and pepper to taste

Directions:
1. Mix beets and spinach in a salad bowl.
2. Add in yogurt, horseradish, and vinegar. You can also add salt and pepper if you wish.
3. Serve the salad as soon as mixed.

Nutrition:
- Calories: 112
- Fat: 11 g
- Fiber: 8 g
- Carbs: 10 g; Protein: 12 g

Olive and Red Bean Salad

Preparation Time: 10 minutes

Cooking Time: 20 minutes

Servings: 4

Ingredients:

- 2 red onions, sliced
- 2 garlic cloves, minced
- 2 tablespoons balsamic vinegar
- 1/4 cup green olives, sliced
- Salt and pepper to taste
- 2 cups mixed greens
- 1 can red beans, drained
- 1 pinch chili flakes
- 2 tablespoons extra-virgin olive oil
- 2 tablespoons parsley, chopped

Directions:

1. In a salad bowl, mix all ingredients
2. Season with salt and pepper, if desired, and serve right away.

Nutrition:

- Calories: 112
- Fat: 11 g
- Fiber: 8 g
- Carbs: 10 g
- Protein: 12 g

Fresh and Light Cabbage Salad

Preparation Time: 10 minutes

Cooking Time: 25 minutes

Servings: 4

Ingredients:

- 1 tablespoon mint, chopped
- 1/2 teaspoon ground coriander
- 1 savoy cabbage, shredded
- 1/2 cup Greek yogurt
- 1/4 teaspoon cumin seeds
- 2 tablespoons extra-virgin olive oil
- 1 carrot, grated
- 1 red onion, sliced
- 1 teaspoon honey
- 1 teaspoon lemon zest
- 2 tablespoons lemon juice
- Salt and pepper to taste

Directions:

1. In a salad bowl, mix all ingredients.
2. You can add salt and pepper to suit your taste and then mix again.
3. This salad is best when cool and freshly made.

Nutrition:

- Calories: 112
- Fat: 11 g
- Fiber: 8 g
- Carbs: 10 g
- Protein: 12 g

Vegetable Patch Salad

Preparation Time: 10 minutes
Cooking Time: 30 minutes
Servings: 6
Ingredients:

- 1 bunch cauliflower, cut into florets
- 1 zucchini, sliced
- 1 sweet potato, peeled and cubed
- 1/2 pounds baby carrots
- Salt and pepper to taste
- 1 teaspoon dried basil
- 2 red onions, sliced
- 2 eggplants, cubed
- 1 endive, sliced
- 3 tablespoons extra-virgin olive oil
- 1 lemon, juiced
- 1 tablespoon balsamic vinegar

Directions:

1. Preheat oven to 350°F. Mix together all vegetables, basil, salt, pepper, and oil in a baking dish and cook for 25-30 minutes.
2. After cooked, pour into a salad bowl and stir in vinegar and lemon juice.
3. Dish up and serve.

Nutrition:

- Calories: 115
- Fat: 9 g
- Fiber: 85 g
- Carbs: 11 g
- Protein: 15 g

Cashews and Red Cabbage Salad

Preparation Time: 10 minutes

Cooking Time: 0 minutes

Servings: 4

Ingredients:
- 1-pound red cabbage, shredded
- 2 tablespoons coriander, chopped
- 1/2 cup cashews halved
- 2 tablespoons olive oil
- 1 tomato, cubed
- A pinch of salt and black pepper
- 1 tablespoon white vinegar

Directions:
1. Mix the cabbage with the coriander and the rest of the ingredients in a salad bowl, toss, and serve cold.

Nutrition:
- Calories: 210
- Fat: 6.3 g
- Protein: 8 g

Apples and Pomegranate Salad

Preparation Time: 10 minutes

Cooking Time: 0 minutes

Servings: 4

Ingredients:

- 3 big apples, cored and cubed
- 1 cup pomegranate seeds
- 3 cups baby arugula
- 1 cup walnuts, chopped
- 1 tablespoon olive oil
- 1 teaspoon white sesame seeds
- 2 tablespoons apple cider vinegar

Directions:

1. Mix the apples with the arugula and the rest of the ingredients in a bowl, toss, and serve cold.

Nutrition:

- Calories: 160
- Fat: 4.3 g
- Protein: 10 g

Cranberry Bulgur Mix

Preparation Time: 10 minutes

Cooking Time: 0 minutes

Servings: 4

Ingredients:

- 1 1/2 cups hot water
- 1 cup bulgur
- Juice of 1/2 lemon
- 4 tablespoons cilantro, chopped
- 1/2 cup cranberries
- 1 1/2 teaspoons curry powder
- 1/4 cup green onions
- 1/2 cup red bell peppers
- 1/2 cup carrots, grated
- 1 tablespoon olive oil

Directions:

1. Put bulgur into a bowl, add the water, stir, cover, leave aside for 10 minutes, fluff, and transfer to a bowl. Merge the rest of the ingredients, toss, and serve cold.

Nutrition:

- Calories: 300
- Fat: 6.4 g
- Protein: 13 g

Chickpeas Corn and Black Beans Salad

Preparation Time: 10 minutes

Cooking Time: 0 minutes

Servings: 4

Ingredients:
- 1 1/2 cups black beans
- 1/2 teaspoon garlic powder
- 2 teaspoons chili powder
- 1 1/2 cups canned chickpeas
- 1 cup baby spinach
- 1 avocado, pitted, peeled, and chopped
- 1 cup corn kernels, chopped
- 2 tablespoons lemon juice
- 1 tablespoon olive oil
- 1 tablespoon apple cider vinegar
- 1 teaspoon chives, chopped

Directions:
1. Mix the black beans with the garlic powder, chili powder, and the rest of the ingredients in a bowl, toss and serve cold.

Nutrition:

- Calories: 300
- Fat: 13.4 g
- Protein: 13 g

Olives and Lentils Salad

Preparation Time: 10 minutes

Cooking Time: 0 minutes

Servings: 2

Ingredients:

- 1/3 cup canned green lentils
- 1 tablespoon olive oil
- 2 cups baby spinach
- 1 cup black olives
- 2 tablespoons sunflower seeds
- 1 tablespoon Dijon mustard
- 2 tablespoons balsamic vinegar
- 2 tablespoons olive oil

Directions:

1. Mix the lentils with the spinach, olives, and the rest of the ingredients in a salad bowl, toss and serve cold.

Nutrition:

- Calories: 279
- Fat: 6.5 g
- Protein: 12 g

Lime Spinach and Chickpeas Salad

Preparation Time: 10 minutes

Cooking Time: 0 minutes

Servings: 4

Ingredients:

- 16 ounces canned chickpeas
- 2 cups baby spinach leaves
- 1/2 tablespoon lime juice
- 2 tablespoons olive oil
- 1 teaspoon cumin, ground
- 1/2 teaspoon chili flakes

Directions:

1. Mix the chickpeas with the spinach and the rest of the ingredients in a large bowl, toss, and serve cold.

Nutrition:

- Calories: 240
- Fat: 8.2 g
- Protein: 12 g

Minty Olives and Tomatoes Salad

Preparation Time: 10 minutes

Cooking Time: 0 minutes

Servings: 4

Ingredients:

- 1 cup kalamata olives
- 1 cup black olives
- 1 cup cherry tomatoes
- 4 tomatoes
- 1 red onion, chopped
- 2 tablespoons oregano, chopped
- 1 tablespoon mint, chopped
- 2 tablespoons balsamic vinegar
- 1/4 cup olive oil
- 2 teaspoons Italian herbs, dried

Directions:

1. In a salad bowl, mix the olives with the tomatoes and the rest of the ingredients, toss, and serve cold.

Nutrition:

- Calories: 190
- Fat: 8.1 g ; Protein: 4.6 g

Beans and Cucumber Salad

Preparation Time: 10 minutes

Cooking Time: 0 minutes

Servings: 4

Ingredients:

- 15 ounces canned great northern beans
- 2 tablespoons olive oil
- 1/2 cup baby arugula
- 1 cup cucumber
- 1 tablespoon parsley
- 2 tomatoes, cubed
- 2 tablespoon balsamic vinegar

Directions:

1. Mix the beans with the cucumber and the rest of the ingredients in a large bowl, toss, and serve cold.

Nutrition:

- Calories: 233
- Fat: 9 g
- Protein: 8 g

Tomato and Avocado Salad

Preparation Time: 10 minutes

Cooking Time: 0 minutes

Servings: 4

Ingredients:

- 1-pound cherry tomatoes
- 2 avocados
- 1 sweet onion, chopped
- 2 tablespoons lemon juice
- 1 1/2 tablespoons olive oil
- Handful basil, chopped

Directions:

1. Mix the tomatoes with the avocados and the rest of the ingredients in a serving bowl, toss, and serve right away.

Nutrition:

- Calories: 148
- Fat: 7.8 g
- Protein: 5.5 g

Feta Tomato Salad

Preparation Time: 5 minutes

Cooking Time: 0 minutes

Servings: 4

Ingredients:

- 2 tablespoons balsamic vinegar
- 1 teaspoon freshly minced basil
- 5 teaspoon salt
- 5 cup coarsely chopped sweet onion
- 2 tablespoons olive oil
- 1 pound cherry or grape tomatoes
- 25 cup crumbled feta cheese

Directions:

1. Whisk the salt, basil, and vinegar. Toss the onion into the vinegar mixture for 5 minutes
2. Slice the tomatoes into halves and stir in the tomatoes, feta cheese, and oil to serve.

Nutrition:

- Calories: 121
- Fats: 9 g
- Protein: 3 g

Grilled Vegetable Salad

Preparation Time: 5 minutes
Cooking Time: 7 minutes
Servings: 3
Ingredients:

- ¼ cup extra virgin olive oil, for brushing
- ¼ cup fresh basil leaves
- ¼ lb. feta cheese
- ½ bunch asparagus, trimmed and cut into bite-size pieces
- 1 medium onion, cut into ½ inch rings
- 1-pint cherry tomatoes
- 1 red bell pepper, quartered, seeds and ribs removed
- 1 yellow bell pepper, quartered, seeds and ribs removed
- Pepper and salt to taste

Directions:

1. Toss olive oil and vegetables in a big bowl. Season with salt and pepper.
2. Frill vegetables in a preheated griller for 5-7 minutes or until charred and tender.
3. Transfer veggies to a platter, add feta and basil.
4. In a separate small bowl, mix olive oil, balsamic vinegar, garlic seasoned with pepper and salt.
5. Drizzle dressing over vegetables and serve.

Nutrition:

- Calories: 147.6
- Protein: 3.8g
- Fat: 19.2g; Carbs: 13.9 g

Healthy Detox Salad

Preparation Time: 5 minutes
Cooking Time: 0 minutes
Servings: 4
Ingredients:

- 4 cups mixed greens
- 2 tbsp lemon juice
- 2 tbsp pumpkin seed oil
- 1 tbsp chia seeds
- 2 tbsp almonds, chopped
- 1 large apple, diced
- 1 large carrot, coarsely grated
- 1 large beet, coarsely grated

Directions:

1. In a medium salad bowl, except for mixed greens, combine all ingredients thoroughly.
2. Into 4 salad plates, divide the mixed greens.
3. Evenly top mixed greens with the salad bowl mixture.
4. Serve and enjoy.

Nutrition:

- Calories: 141
- Protein: 2.1g
- Carbs: 14.7g
- Fat: 8.2g

Herbed Calamari Salad

Preparation Time: 10 minutes
Cooking Time: 25 minutes
Servings: 3
Ingredients:

- ¼ cup finely chopped cilantro leaves
- ¼ cup finely chopped mint leaves
- ¼ tsp freshly ground black pepper
- ½ cup finely chopped flat leaf parsley leaves
- ¾ tsp kosher salt
- 2 ½ lbs. cleaned and trimmed uncooked calamari rings and tentacles, defrosted
- 3 medium garlic cloves, smashed and minced
- 3 tbsp extra virgin olive oil
- A pinch of crushed red pepper flakes
- Juice of 1 large lemon
- Peel of 1 lemon, thinly sliced into strips

Directions:

1. On a nonstick large fry pan, heat 1 ½ tbsp olive oil. Once hot, sauté garlic until fragrant around a minute.
2. Add calamari, making sure that they are in one layer, if pan is too small then cook in batches.
3. Season with pepper and salt, after 2 to 4 minutes of searing, remove calamari from pan with a slotted spoon and transfer to a large bowl. Continue cooking remainder of calamari.
4. Season cooked calamari with herbs, lemon rind, lemon juice, red pepper flakes, pepper, salt, and remaining olive oil.
5. Toss well to coat, serve and enjoy.

Nutrition:

- Calories: 551.7
- Protein: 7.3g
- Carbs: 121.4g
- Fat: 4.1g

Herbed Chicken Salad Greek Style

Preparation Time: 5 minutes

Cooking Time: 0 minutes

Servings: 6

Ingredients:

- ¼ cup or 1 oz crumbled feta cheese
- ½ tsp garlic powder
- ½ tsp salt
- ¾ tsp black pepper, divided
- 1 cup grape tomatoes, halved
- 1 cup peeled and chopped English cucumbers
- 1 cup plain fat-free yogurt
- 1 pound skinless, boneless chicken breast, cut into 1-inch cubes
- 1 tsp bottled minced garlic
- 1 tsp ground oregano
- 2 tsp sesame seed paste or tahini
- 5 tsp fresh lemon juice, divided
- 6 pitted kalamata olives, halved
- 8 cups chopped romaine lettuce
- Cooking spray

Directions:

1. In a bowl, mix together ¼ tsp salt, ½ tsp pepper, garlic powder and oregano. Then on medium high heat place a skillet and coat with cooking spray and sauté together the spice mixture and chicken until chicken is cooked. Before transferring to bowl, drizzle with juice.
2. In a small bowl, mix thoroughly the following: garlic, tahini, yogurt, ¼ tsp pepper, ¼ tsp salt, and 2 tsp juice.

3. In another bowl, mix together olives, tomatoes, cucumber and lettuce.
4. To Serve salad, place 2 ½ cups of lettuce mixture on plate, topped with ½ cup chicken mixture, 3 tbsp yogurt mixture and 1 tbsp of cheese.

Nutrition:

- Calories: 170.1
- Fat: 3.7g
- Protein: 20.7g
- Carbs: 13.5g

Mediterranean Chicken Salad

Preparation Time: 5 minutes
Cooking Time: 25 minutes
Servings: 4
Ingredients:

- For Chicken:
- 1 ¾ lb. boneless, skinless chicken breast
- ¼ teaspoon each of pepper and salt (or as desired)
- 1 ½ tablespoon of butter, melted
- For Mediterranean salad:
- 1 cup of sliced cucumber
- 6 cups of romaine lettuce, that is torn or roughly chopped
- 10 pitted Kalamata olives
- 1 pint of cherry tomatoes
- 1/3 cup of reduced-fat feta cheese
- ¼ teaspoon each of pepper and salt (or lesser)
- 1 small lemon juice (it should be about 2 tablespoons)

Directions:

1. Preheat your oven or grill to about 350F. Season the chicken with salt, butter, and black pepper. Roast or grill chicken until it reaches an internal temperature of 1650F in about 25 minutes.
2. Once your chicken breasts are cooked, remove and keep aside to rest for about 5 minutes before you slice it.
3. Combine all the salad ingredients you have and toss everything together very well. Serve the chicken with Mediterranean salad.

Nutrition:

- Calories: 340 ; Protein: 45g ; Carbohydrate: 9g ; Fat: 4 g

Shrimp Salad Cocktails

Preparation Time: 35 minutes
Cooking Time: 35 minutes
Servings: 8
Ingredients:

- 2 cups mayonnaise
- 6 plum tomatoes, seeded and finely chopped
- 1/4 cup ketchup
- 1/4 cup lemon juice
- 2 cups seedless red and green grapes, halved
- 1 tablespoon. Worcestershire sauce
- 2 lbs. peeled and deveined cooked large shrimp
- 2 celery ribs, finely chopped
- 3 tablespoons. minced fresh tarragon or 3 teaspoon dried tarragon
- salt and 1/4 teaspoon pepper
- shredded 2 of cups romaine
- papaya or 1/2 cup peeled chopped mango
- parsley or minced chives

Directions:

1. Combine Worcestershire sauce, lemon juice, ketchup and mayonnaise together in a small bowl. Combine pepper, salt, tarragon, celery and shrimp together in a large bowl.
2. Put in 1 cup of dressing toss well to coat. Scoop 1 tablespoon. of the dressing into 8 cocktail glasses.
3. Layer each glass with 1/4 cup of lettuce, followed by 1/2 cup of the shrimp mixture, 1/4 cup of grapes, 1/3 cup of tomatoes and finally 1 tablespoon. of mango.

4. Spread the remaining dressing over top; sprinkle chives on top. Serve immediately.

Nutrition:

- Calories: 580
- Carbohydrate: 16 g
- Fat: 46 g
- Protein: 24 g

Garlic Chive Cauliflower Mash

Preparation Time: 20 minutes
Cooking Time: 18 minutes
Servings: 5
Ingredients:

- 4 cups cauliflower
- 1/3 cup vegetarian mayonnaise
- 1 garlic clove
- 1/2 teaspoon. kosher salt
- 1 tablespoon. water
- 1/8 teaspoon. pepper
- 1/4 teaspoon. lemon juice
- 1/2 teaspoon lemon zest
- 1 tablespoon Chives, minced

Directions:

1. In a bowl that is save to microwave, add the cauliflower, mayo, garlic, water, and salt/pepper and mix until the cauliflower is well coated. Cook on high for 15-18 minutes, until the cauliflower is almost mushy.
2. Blend the mixture in a strong blender until completely smooth, adding a little more water if the mixture is too chunky. Season with the remaining ingredients and serve.

Nutrition:

- Calories: 178
- Carbohydrate: 14 g
- Fat: 18 g
- Protein: 2 g

Beet Greens with Pine Nuts Goat Cheese

Preparation Time: 25 minutes

Cooking Time: 15 minutes

Servings: 3

Ingredients:

- 4 cups beet tops, washed and chopped roughly
- 1 teaspoon. EVOO
- 1 tablespoon. no sugar added balsamic vinegar
- 2 oz. crumbled dry goat cheese
- 2 tablespoons. Toasted pine nuts

Directions:

1. Warm the oil in a pan, then cook the beet greens on medium high heat until they release their moisture. Let it cook until almost tender.
2. Flavor with salt and pepper and remove from heat. Toss the greens in a mixture of balsamic vinegar and olive oil, then top with the nuts and cheese. Serve warm.

Nutrition:

- Calories: 215
- Carbohydrate: 4 g
- Fat: 18 g
- Protein: 10 g

Kale Slaw and Strawberry Salad + Poppyseed Dressing

Preparation Time: 10 minutes
Cooking Time: 20 minutes
Servings: 2
Ingredients:

- Chicken breast; 8 ounces; sliced and baked
- Kale; 1 cup; chopped
- Slaw mix; 1 cup (cabbage, broccoli slaw, carrots mixed)
- Slivered almonds; 1/4 cup
- Strawberries; 1 cup; sliced
- For the dressing:
- Light mayonnaise; 1 tablespoon
- Dijon mustard
- Olive oil; 1 tablespoon
- Apple cider vinegar; 1 tablespoon
- Lemon juice; 1/2 teaspoon
- 1 tablespoon of honey
- Onion powder; 1/4 teaspoon
- Garlic powder; 1/4 teaspoon
- Poppyseeds

Directions:

1. Whisk the dressing ingredients together until well mixed, then leave to cool in the fridge. Slice the chicken breasts.
2. Divide 2 bowls of spinach, slaw, and strawberries. Cover with a sliced breast of chicken (4 oz. each), then scatter with almonds. Divide the dressing between the two bowls and drizzle.

Nutrition:

- Calories: 150
- Carbs: 17g
- Fat: 1g
- Protein: 7g

Spring Greek Salad

Preparation Time: 15 minutes
Cooking Time: 0 minutes
Servings: 4
Ingredients:

- 1 head escarole, chopped
- 1 head curly chicory, chopped
- ¼ cup crumbled feta cheese
- ¼ cup pitted halved kalamata olives
- ¼ cup sliced seeded pepperoncini
- 3 tablespoons extra-virgin olive oil
- Juice of ½ lemon
- 2 garlic cloves, minced
- Pinch dried dill
- Salt
- Freshly ground black pepper

Directions:

1. In a large bowl, toss together the escarole and chicory. Scatter the feta cheese, olives, and pepperoncini on top.
2. In a small bowl, whisk together the olive oil, lemon juice, and garlic. Season with the dill and salt and pepper to taste. Pour the dressing over the lettuce mixture and toss to combine.

Nutrition:

- Calories: 173
- Fat: 14g
- Protein: 5g
- Carbohydrates: 10g

Panzanella

Preparation Time: 15 minutes
Cooking Time: 10 minutes
Servings: 6
Ingredients:

- ¼ cup extra-virgin olive oil, plus 3 tablespoons
- 6 stale hearty Italian bread slices, cut into cubes
- 6 tomatoes, cut into 1-inch pieces
- 1 cucumber, halved lengthwise and cut into half-moons
- 1 red bell pepper, seeded and finely chopped
- ½ onion, thinly sliced
- 2 tablespoons roughly chopped capers
- 2 tablespoons red wine vinegar
- 1 garlic clove, minced
- 1 teaspoon salt
- ¼ teaspoon freshly ground black pepper
- 1 teaspoon chopped fresh basil

Directions:

1. In a large skillet, heat 3 tablespoons of olive oil over medium heat. Add the bread cubes and cook for about 10 minutes, until browned on all sides.
2. Transfer the bread cubes to a large bowl and add the tomatoes, cucumber, bell pepper, onion, and capers.
3. In a small bowl, whisk together the remaining ¼ cup of olive oil, the vinegar, garlic, salt, and pepper. Pour the dressing over the salad and toss to combine well.
4. Let the salad rest for 30 minutes. Sprinkle the basil on top and serve.

Nutrition:

- Calories: 205
- Fat: 17g
- Protein: 3g
- Carbohydrates: 13g

Tuscan Tuna Salad

Preparation Time: 15 minutes
Cooking Time: 0 minutes
Servings: 4
Ingredients:

- ¼ cup extra-virgin olive oil
- Juice of ½ lemon
- ½ teaspoon Dijon mustard
- Salt
- Freshly ground black pepper
- 2 (5-ounce) cans tuna in olive oil, drained
- 1 (19-ounce) can cannellini beans, rinsed and drained
- 12 marinated mushrooms, rinsed and halved if large
- 12 grape or cherry tomatoes, halved
- 1 or 2 celery stalks, sliced
- 1 teaspoon capers (optional)

Directions:

1. In a small bowl, whisk together the olive oil, lemon juice, and mustard, and season with salt and pepper.
2. In a large bowl, combine the tuna, beans, mushrooms, tomatoes, celery, and capers (if using). Add the dressing and toss well. Season with additional salt and pepper, if desired.

Nutrition:

- Calories: 389
- Fat: 20g
- Protein: 26g
- Carbohydrates: 29g

Mediterranean Chopped Salad

Preparation Time: 15 minutes

Cooking Time: 20 minutes

Servings: 4

Ingredients:

- 1 cup whole grains, such as red or white quinoa, millet, or buckwheat
- 1 (15-ounce) can chickpeas, rinsed and drained
- 2 cups baby spinach
- 1 cucumber, finely chopped
- ½ red bell pepper, finely chopped
- ½ fennel bulb, trimmed and finely chopped
- 1 celery stalk, finely chopped
- 1 carrot, finely chopped
- 1 plum tomato, finely chopped
- ½ red onion, finely chopped
- 1 cherry pepper, seeded and finely chopped
- ¼ cup extra-virgin olive oil
- 2 tablespoons white wine vinegar
- 1 teaspoon chopped fresh basil
- 1 garlic clove, minced
- Salt
- Freshly ground black pepper

Directions:

1. Cook the whole grains according to package directions. Allow to cool. In a large bowl, toss the grains, chickpeas, spinach, cucumber, bell pepper, fennel, celery, carrot, tomato, red onion, and cherry pepper.
2. In a small bowl, whisk together the olive oil, vinegar, basil, and garlic. Season with salt and pepper. Toss with the salad and serve.

Nutrition:

- Calories: 401
- Fat: 18g
- Protein: 12g
- Carbohydrates: 50g

Green Bean and Potato Salad

Preparation Time: 15 minutes
Cooking Time: 15 minutes
Servings: 4
Ingredients:

- 2 russet potatoes, peeled and cut into 1-inch pieces
- 2 cups green beans, trimmed
- ¼ cup extra-virgin olive oil
- Juice of ½ lemon
- 1 teaspoon Italian Herb Blend
- 1 teaspoon salt
- ½ teaspoon freshly ground black pepper

Directions:

1. Put the potatoes in a saucepan, cover with water, and bring to a boil over high heat. Cook for about 10 minutes, until tender. Drain and set aside to cool.
2. While the potatoes are cooling, fill the same saucepan with water and bring to a boil over high heat. Fill a large bowl with ice cubes and cold water.
3. Add the green beans to the boiling water and blanch for about 3 minutes, then remove with tongs or a sieve and immediately plunge them into the ice bath. Once cool, drain.
4. Combine the potatoes and green beans in a large bowl. Drizzle the olive oil over the vegetables and squeeze in the lemon juice. Add the Italian herb blend, salt, and pepper and toss to combine.

Nutrition:

- Calories: 282; Fat: 14g ; Protein: 5g ; Carbohydrates: 37g

Shrimp Salad

Preparation Time: 15 minutes
Cooking Time: 5 minutes
Servings: 4
Ingredients:

- 1-pound large shrimp, peeled and deveined
- Juice of ½ lemon
- 2 celery stalks, chopped
- 3 scallions, chopped
- 1 garlic clove, minced
- Salt
- Freshly ground black pepper
- ½ cup vegan mayonnaise

Directions:

1. Put the shrimp in a skillet and add a few tablespoons of water. Cook over medium heat for 2 to 3 minutes, until the shrimp turn pink. Drain and pat dry. Cut the shrimp into bite-size pieces and transfer a bowl.
2. Add the lemon juice and toss, then add the celery, scallions, and garlic. Season with salt and pepper. Toss again to combine. Add the vegan mayonnaise and fold gently to combine.

Nutrition:

- Calories: 185
- Fat: 11g
- Protein: 18g
- Carbohydrates: 4g

Warm Potato Salad

Preparation Time: 15 minutes
Cooking Time: 10 minutes
Servings: 4
Ingredients:

- 6 red potatoes, cut into 1-inch pieces
- 1 tablespoon white wine vinegar
- 3 large eggs, hard-boiled, peeled, and chopped
- 2 celery stalks, finely chopped
- 1 small onion, finely chopped
- ½ cup mayonnaise or vegan mayonnaise
- 1 teaspoon Dijon mustard
- 1 teaspoon salt
- ¼ teaspoon freshly ground black pepper

Directions:

1. Put the potatoes in a saucepan, cover with water, and bring to a boil over high heat. Cook for about 10 minutes, until tender. Drain and transfer to a large bowl, then sprinkle with the vinegar.
2. Add the eggs, celery, and onion and toss. Add the mayonnaise, mustard, salt, and pepper and toss to combine. Serve.

Nutrition:

- Calories: 474
- Fat: 25g
- Protein: 11g
- Carbohydrates: 53g

Summer Rainbow Salad

Preparation Time: 15 minutes
Cooking Time: 0 minutes
Servings: 4
Ingredients:

- 1 cup chopped red or green leaf lettuce
- 1 cup chopped iceberg lettuce
- ½ cup baby arugula
- ½ cup chopped radicchio
- 1 cup mixed chopped or sliced vegetables, such as red cabbage, red onion, radish, red or yellow tomato, carrot, cucumber, and avocado
- ¼ cup extra-virgin olive oil
- Juice of ½ lemon
- ½ teaspoon salt
- ¼ teaspoon freshly ground black pepper
- ¼ teaspoon dried oregano

Directions:

1. In a large salad bowl, combine the lettuces, arugula, radicchio, and mixed vegetables and gently toss.
2. In a small bowl, whisk together the olive oil, lemon juice, salt, pepper, and oregano. Pour the dressing over the salad and toss well to coat.

Nutrition:

- Calories: 137
- Fat: 14g
- Protein: 1g ; Carbohydrates: 4g

Arugula and White Bean Salad

Preparation Time: 15 minutes

Cooking Time: 0 minutes

Servings: 2

Ingredients:

- 1 (15-ounce) can cannellini beans, rinsed and drained
- 2 cups baby arugula
- ¼ cup extra-virgin olive oil
- Juice of ½ lemon
- ½ teaspoon dried oregano
- ½ teaspoon salt
- ¼ teaspoon freshly ground black pepper
- 4 Italian seeded bread slices, toasted

Directions:

1. In a medium bowl, combine the beans and arugula. In a small bowl, whisk together the olive oil, lemon juice, oregano, salt, and pepper. Pour over the salad and toss to coat.
2. To serve, spoon heaping portions of the salad over the toast.

Nutrition:

- Calories: 469
- Fat: 29g
- Protein: 14g
- Carbohydrates: 42g

Fennel and Orange Salad

Preparation Time: 15 minutes

Cooking Time: 0 minutes

Servings: 6

Ingredients:

- 4 navel oranges, peeled, halved, and thinly sliced
- 3 fennel bulbs, trimmed and thinly sliced, fronds reserved for garnish
- 2 tablespoons extra-virgin olive oil
- 1 tablespoon white wine vinegar
- Salt
- Freshly ground black pepper

Directions:

1. In a large bowl, combine the orange and fennel slices. In a small bowl, whisk together the olive oil and vinegar. Season with salt and pepper.
2. Pour the dressing over the orange and fennel and toss to combine. Roughly chop the fennel fronds and sprinkle them on top.

Nutrition: Calories: 122 Fat: 5g Protein: 2g Carbohydrates: 20g

Grilled Mahi-Mahi with Jicama Slaw

Preparation Time: 20 minutes
Cooking Time: 10 minutes
Servings: 4
Ingredients:

- 1 teaspoon each for pepper and salt, divided
- 1 tablespoon of lime juice, divided
- 2 tablespoon + 2 teaspoons of extra virgin olive oil
- 4 raw mahi-mahi fillets, which should be about 8 oz. each
- ½ cucumber which should be thinly cut into long strips (it should yield about 1 cup)
- 1 jicama, which should be thinly cut into long strips (it should yield about 3 cups)
- 1 cup of alfalfa sprouts
- 2 cups of coarsely chopped watercress

Directions:

1. Combine ½ teaspoon of both pepper and salt, 1 teaspoon of lime juice, and 2 teaspoons of oil in a small bowl. Then brush the mahi-mahi fillets all through with the olive oil mixture.
2. Grill the mahi-mahi on medium-high heat until it becomes done in about 5 minutes, turn it to the other side, and let it be done for about 5 minutes.
3. For the slaw, combine the watercress, cucumber, jicama, and alfalfa sprouts in a bowl. Now combine ½ teaspoon of both pepper and salt, 2 teaspoons of lime juice, and 2 tablespoons of extra virgin oil in a small bowl. Drizzle it over slaw and toss together to combine.

Nutrition:

- Calories: 320
- Protein: 44g
- Carbohydrate: 10g
- Fat: 11 g

Lightning Source UK Ltd.
Milton Keynes UK
UKHW020640270521
384471UK00010B/785